Paleo Diet
Beginners Cookbook

100 Easy & Creative
Paleo Recipes for Beginners

Mark Daily

Printed in The United States of America

First Printing, 2013

Salem Fox Press

www.salemfox.com

Table of Contents

INTRODUCTION

If you're just getting started on a Paleo diet, many of the recipes can be daunting. From food processors to ingredients that will require more energy to hunt down than they'll give you in return, many Paleo recipes are a lot of work.

Paleo Diet Beginners Cookbook is jam-packed with easy recipes for those who are new to the Paleo diet and are ready to get started making delicious, ultra-healthful recipes fast.

From breakfast in the morning to dessert in the evening, we've got you covered with tons of recipes for every step of the way.

BREAKFAST

Apple Bacon Omelette

Ingredients
1 apple
3 slices of bacon
2 eggs
1/2 tsp. olive oil
Sea salt and ground pepper to taste

Directions
1. Put the bacon in a non-stick pan and set to medium heat. Heat for about 10 minutes or until bacon is a deep brown color.
2. While your bacon is cooking, crack the eggs into a medium bowl and stir them up. Dice up some apples and set them aside.
3. When your bacon is done cooking, take it out of the pan and set it aside.
4. Pour the olive oil and the eggs into the pan you just used to cook the bacon. Don't pour out the bacon fat - it gives the omelette extra flavor.
5. Tilt the pan around so that the eggs evenly fill up the center of the pan.
6. Season the eggs with a dash of salt and pepper.

(continued on next page)

7. When your eggs start to look like a firm, bright yellow pancake, flip them over with a spatula.
8. Crumble your bacon and spoon your diced apples and bacon in a straight line in the center of the eggs.
9. Lift one side of the eggs and fold it over. Transfer to a plate. Serve.

Servings: 1

Blueberry Walnut Omelette

Ingredients
1/4 cup blueberries
2 Tablespoons walnuts
2 eggs
1/2 tsp. olive oil
Sea salt and ground pepper to taste

Directions
1. Pour the olive oil into a pan and set to medium heat. Allow the oil to get hot · about 4 minutes.
2. Crack the eggs into a small bowl and stir.
3. Pour the eggs into the pan.
4. Tilt the pan around so the eggs evenly fill up the center of the pan.
5. Season the eggs with a dash of salt and pepper.
6. When your eggs start to look like a firm, bright yellow pancake, flip them over with a spatula.
7. Drop your blueberries and walnuts in a straight line in the center of the eggs.
8. Lift one side of the eggs and fold it over. Transfer to a plate. Serve.

Servings: 1

Bacon Egg Muffins

Ingredients
4 slices of bacon
4 eggs
1 tsp. olive oil
Sea salt and pepper to taste

Directions
1. Preheat the oven to 375.
2. Put the bacon in a non-stick pan and set to medium heat. Heat for about 3 minutes, because you only want to partially cook the bacon. Then take it out of the pan and set it aside.
3. Brush olive oil into four of the muffin cups in a muffin pan.
4. Using one slice of bacon for each cup, wrap the inside of each muffin cup with the bacon to make a ring.
5. Crack one egg into each bacon-lined muffin cup. Season with salt and pepper.
6. Bake the bacon egg muffins for 10-15 minutes or until set. Transfer to a plate. Serve.

Servings: Makes 4 Bacon Egg Muffins

Salmon & Avocado Scrambled Eggs

Ingredients
3/4 cup cooked smoked salmon
1 avocado
4 eggs
1 tsp. olive oil
Sea salt and pepper to taste

Directions
1. Pour the olive oil in a pan and allow it to get hot - about 4 minutes.
2. Crack the eggs directly into the hot pan and stir.
3. Crumble the salmon and drop into the uncooked eggs. Mix the eggs and salmon thoroughly. Season with salt and pepper.
4. Dice avocado and set it aside.
5. Cook eggs and salmon for 3-4 minutes, or until eggs are set.
6. Turn off the heat and toss in the diced avocados. Transfer to a plate. Serve.

Servings: 2

Maple Burger Scrambled Eggs

Ingredients
3/4 cup cooked ground beef
1/4 cup maple syrup
4 eggs
1 tsp. olive oil
Sea salt and pepper to taste

Directions
1. Pour the olive oil in a pan and allow it to get hot ·· about 4 minutes.
2. Crack the eggs directly into the hot pan and stir. Stir in ground beef and maple syrup. Season with salt and pepper.
3. Cook for about 3·4 minutes, or until eggs are set. Transfer to a plate. Serve.

Servings: 2

Maple Blueberry Scrambled Eggs

Ingredients
1/4 cup maple syrup
1/2 cup blueberries
4 eggs
1 tsp. olive oil
Sea salt and pepper to taste

Directions
1. Pour the olive oil in a pan and allow it to get hot -- about 4 minutes.
2. Crack the eggs directly into the hot pan and stir. Stir in blueberries and maple syrup. Season with salt and pepper.
3. Cook for about 3-4 minutes, or until eggs are set. Transfer to a plate. Serve.

Servings: 2

Sweet Potato Scrambled Eggs

Ingredients
1 small sweet potato
2 eggs
1 Tablespoon olive oil
Sea salt and pepper to taste

Directions
1. Pour the olive oil in a pan and allow it to get hot - about 4 minutes.
2. While the oil is heating up, clean the sweet potato and dice it into small cubes. Throw the sweet potato into the hot oil and let it fry for 2-3 minutes. Crack the eggs into the pan with the sweet potatoes and stir. Season with salt and pepper.
3. Cook for 3-4 minutes, or until eggs are set. Transfer to a plate. Serve.

Servings: 1

Roasted Blueberries & Macadamia Nuts

Ingredients
1 cup blueberries
1 Tablespoon honey
1/2 cup macadamia nuts

Directions
1. Set the oven to 400 degrees.
2. Spread the macadamia nuts out on a baking sheet and cook for 20 minutes.
3. Take out the baking sheet and mix the blueberries with the nuts. Drizzle honey over blueberries and nuts.
4. Cook for an additional 10 minutes.
Transfer to a bowl. Serve.

Servings: 2

Crispy Kale & Bacon Omelette

Ingredients
1 cup of kale
3 slices of bacon
2 eggs
1 tsp. olive oil
Sea salt and ground pepper to taste

Directions
1. Pour half the olive oil into a pan and set to medium heat. Allow the oil to get hot · about 4 minutes.
2. Drop kale into the hot oil. Season with salt and pepper.
3. Move kale around with tongs so it doesn't burn. Cook for two minutes.
4. Put the bacon in a separate pan and set to medium heat. Heat for about 10 minutes or until bacon is a deep brown color.
5. When the bacon is done cooking, take it out of the pan and set it aside.
6. Crack your eggs into a bowl and stir them up. Then pour them into the hot pan you just used to cook the bacon. Don't pour out the bacon fat · it gives the omelette extra flavor.

(continued on next page)

7. Tilt the pan around so that the eggs evenly fill up the center of the pan.
Season the eggs with a dash of salt and pepper.
8. When your eggs start to look like a firm, bright yellow pancake, flip them over with a spatula.
9. Crumble your bacon and spoon your kale and bacon in a straight line in the center of the eggs.
10. Lift one side of the eggs and fold it over. Transfer to a plate. Serve.

Servings: 1

Nutty Sweet Potato Breakfast Pudding

Ingredients
1 medium sweet potato
1 Tablespoon maple syrup
1/4 cup crushed macadamia nuts

Directions
The Night Before:
1. Set the oven to 400 degrees.
2. Poke some holes into the sweet potato with a fork. Put the sweet potato on a baking sheet and cook for an hour. Take it out and put it on a plate to let it cool for the morning.

The Next Morning:
1. Put the sweet potato in a blender or food processor and puree.
2. Spoon the sweet potatoes in a bowl. Top with crushed macadamia nuts and maple syrup. Serve.

Servings: 2

Avocado Bacon Stuffed Eggs

Ingredients
4 eggs
1 avocado
4 slices of bacon

Directions
1. Set the eggs in a large pot and cover with water. The tops of the eggs should be covered with at least an inch and a half of water. Bring the water to a rolling boil.
2. Take the pot off the heat and cover the top. Let it stand for 14 minutes.
3. While the eggs are cooking, put the bacon on a pan set at medium heat and cook for 10 minutes or until bacon is a deep brown color. Put the bacon on a plate and set aside.
4. Remove the eggs from the pot and peel them under cold running water. Cut the eggs lengthwise in half. Scoop the yolk from the eggs and put it in a medium bowl.
5. Scoop out the avocado and put it in the bowl with the egg yolks. Crumble the bacon and put it in the bowl with the egg yolks and avocado. Stir the egg yolk, avocado, and bacon mixture.

(continued on next page)

6. Scoop the yolk, avocado, and bacon mixture into the egg halves. Serve.

Servings: Makes 8 Avocado Bacon Stuffed Egg Halves

LUNCH

Berry Nutty Salad

Ingredients
2 cups kale
1 cup arugula
1/2 cup blueberries
1/2 cup blackberries
1 cup strawberries
1/4 cup macadamia nuts
1/4 cup walnuts

Directions
1. Mix all ingredients together in a large bowl. Serve.

Servings: 3

Spicy Avocado & Bacon Wrap

Ingredients
2 large romaine leaves
1 avocado
3 slices of bacon
1/2 cup tomatoes
1 Tablespoon of chopped jalapeños

Directions
1. Put the bacon in a non-stick pan and set to medium heat. Heat for about 10 minutes or until bacon is a deep brown color. Take it out of the pan and set aside.
2. Slice avocado and dice tomatoes.
3. Fill lettuce leaves with bacon, avocado, jalapeños, and tomatoes. Roll up the wrap. Serve.

Servings: 1

Salmon Avocado Lime Wrap

Ingredients
2 large romaine leaves
1 avocado
1/2 cup cooked smoked salmon
1/2 cup tomatoes
1 tsp. of lime juice

Directions
1. Slice avocado and dice tomatoes.
2. Fill lettuce leaves with salmon, avocado, and tomatoes. Drizzle with lime juice. Roll up the wrap. Serve.

Servings: 1

Salsa BLT Cups

Ingredients
4 slices of bacon
1 tsp. olive oil
1 cup chopped romaine lettuce
1/2 cup salsa

Directions
1. Preheat the oven to 375.
2. Put the bacon in a non-stick pan and set to medium heat. Heat for about 3 minutes, because you only want to partially cook the bacon. Then take it out of the pan and set it aside.
3. Brush olive oil into four of the muffin cups in a muffin pan.
4. Using one slice of bacon for each cup, wrap the inside of each muffin cup with the bacon to make a ring.
5. Put the muffin pan in the oven for 10 minutes or until bacon is crispy.
6. Fill bacon cups with lettuce and salsa. Transfer to a plate. Serve.

Servings: Makes 4 BLT Cups

Lemon Pepper Tuna Portobellos

Ingredients
1 large portobello mushroom
1 can of tuna
Lemon pepper seasoning to taste

Directions
1. Preheat the oven to 375.
2. Rinse the portobello mushroom and pat dry.
3. Place the mushroom top down onto a baking sheet. Scoop the tuna into the mushroom. Season with lemon pepper.
4. Bake for 8-9 minutes. Transfer to a plate. Serve.

Servings: 1

Bacon Asparagus Wrapped Salmon

Ingredients
4 medium smoked salmon fillets
8 pieces of bacon
8 fresh asparagus spears
2 Tablespoons minced shallots
Olive oil
Pepper to taste

Directions
1. Preheat oven to 375. Wrap each slice of bacon around each asparagus spear.
2. Place the bacon wrapped asparagus on a wax paper. Sprinkle with pepper.
3. Place the smoked salmon fillets on a baking sheet. Top with minced shallots and two bacon wrapped asparagus spears per salmon fillet. Don't overlap the spears.
4. Bake in the oven for 17 minutes. Transfer to a plate. Serve.

Servings: 4

Apple Bacon Salmon Patties

Ingredients
15 oz. can of salmon
1 small diced apple
4 slices of bacon

Directions
1. Put the bacon in a non-stick pan and set to medium heat. Heat for about 10 minutes or until bacon is a deep brown color.
2. While your bacon is cooking, mix the salmon and apples together in a medium bowl.
3. When the bacon has finished cooking, crumble it into the bowl with the salmon and apples.
4. Mash the salmon, apples, and bacon into two patties using your hands.
5. Heat on a non-stick pan over medium heat for 4 minutes, then flip the patties and cook for an additional 4 minutes.

Servings: 2

Garlic Lime Salmon Patties

Ingredients
15 oz. can of salmon
1 Tablespoon minced garlic
1 Tablespoon lime juice
1/2 cup chopped celery

Directions
1. Mix the salmon, garlic, lime, and celery together in a medium bowl. Mash the mixture into two patties using your hands.
2. Heat on a non-stick pan over medium heat for 4 minutes, then flip the patties and cook for an additional 4 minutes.

Servings: 2

Halibut Cucumber Bites

Ingredients
2 halibut fillets
1 Tablespoon minced garlic
1 Tablespoon minced shallots
1/2 tsp. lemon juice
1 medium cucumber, sliced

Directions
1. Preheat oven to 350.
2. Chop the halibut fillets into small pieces and toss into a bowl. Add garlic, shallots, and lemon to the bowl and stir thoroughly.
3. Top cucumber slices with halibut mixture.
4. Bake for 9 minutes. Transfer to a plate. Serve.

Servings: 2

Sweet & Crunchy Apple Turkey Wrap

Ingredients
1/2 sliced apple
2 slices of turkey
1 large romaine lettuce leaf

Directions
1. Set the sliced turkey on top of the romaine leaf. Set the apple slices inside the center of the turkey. Roll up the wrap. Serve.

Servings: 1

Bacon & Onion Stuffed Peaches

Ingredients
1 peach
4 slices of cooked bacon
1 1/2 Tablespoons minced green onion
1 tsp. ground black pepper

Directions
1. Preheat oven to 375.
2. Slice peach in half and remove pit. Scoop peach meat from the shells and put it in a medium bowl. Mash the peach meat.
3. Crumble the bacon and toss in the bowl with the mashed peach. Stir in green onion and black pepper.
4. Scoop peach and bacon mixture into peach shells. Set stuffed peaches, cut side up, on a baking sheet. Bake for 15 minutes. Serve.

Servings: 2

Key Lime Fish Tacos

Ingredients
2 halibut fillets
4 large romaine lettuce leaves
1 Tablespoon minced shallots
1 Tablespoon lime juice
1 diced avocado
1 cup chopped cabbage
1 tsp. ground black pepper
1/2 cup Pineapple Salsa (Recipe included in this book)

Directions
1. Preheat oven to 350.
2. Chop the halibut fillets into small pieces and toss into a bowl. Add lime juice, shallots, and black pepper to the bowl and stir thoroughly.
3. Place the halibut fillets on a baking sheet. Bake halibut fillets for 9 minutes.
4. Fill the four lettuce leaves with the halibut mixture, avocado, cabbage, and pineapple salsa. Serve.

Servings: 4

Bacon Wrapped Sushi

Ingredients
8 slices bacon
1/4 cup crab meat
1/4 cup diced shrimp
1 avocado
1 tsp. lime juice

Directions
1. Put the bacon in a non-stick pan and set to medium heat. Heat for about 10 minutes or until bacon is a deep brown color. Set aside.
2. Mix the crab meat, shrimp, lime juice, and avocado in a bowl.
3. Wrap each slice of bacon tightly around a ball of the crab and avocado mixture. Serve.

Servings: 8

Tuna Salad in Cucumber Cups

Directions
1 medium cucumber
Salt to taste
1 (5 oz.) can tuna, drained
1 Tablespoons minced red onion
1 tsp. olive oil
Ground pepper to taste

Ingredients
1. Cut ends off cucumber. Halve the long way
and scoop out all seeds with a tsp.. Cut the
halves into 2 pieces, sprinkle with salt and
set aside on a plate.
2. In a small bowl combine the tuna, onion,
olive oil and pepper. Carefully scoop tuna
mixture into cucumber cups and serve.

Makes 1 serving

Roasted Cauliflower Soup

Ingredients
1 medium head cauliflower
1 Tablespoon light olive oil
Salt and pepper to taste
1 ½ cups almond milk, warmed
¼ cup toasted sliced almonds

Directions
1. Preheat the oven to 375 degrees F.
2. Remove leaves and tough core from cauliflower and slice florets so they lay flat on a baking sheet. Drizzle the olive oil over, season with salt and pepper, and roast in the oven, occasionally turning florets, until lightly golden on the edges and fork tender, 15 to 20 minutes.
3. Transfer to a food processor, add the warmed almond milk and process until smooth but chunky, adding more milk if desired. For a smoother result, process in a blender on the puree setting.
4. Taste for additional seasoning and serve warm topped with the toasted almonds.

Makes 4 servings

Chicken & Roasted Peppers in Lettuce Wraps

Ingredients
3 to 4 lettuce leaves for wrapping, such as
Boston or leaf lettuce
4 oz. grilled chicken breast, sliced
½ cup roasted red pepper slices (pimentos)
¼ cup fresh basil leaves, torn
Salt and pepper to taste

Directions
1. Lay the lettuce leaves flat on a work
surface. Distribute the chicken and pimento
evenly down the middle of each leaf.
2. Top with the basil and season with salt
and pepper. Carefully fold up the stem end of
the leaf and roll to enclose. Serve
immediately.

Makes 1 serving

Chicken BLT Wedge Salad

Ingredients
1 Wedge (1/4 head) iceberg lettuce
4 slices bacon, fried crisp and crumbled
1 medium tomato, diced

For Dressing:

½ medium avocado, peeled, seeded and
chopped
2 Tablespoons lemon juice
2 Tablespoons unsweetened coconut cream
¼ cup olive oil
2 Tablespoons fresh parsley leaves
Salt and pepper to taste

1. Place the wedge on a serving plate. Top
with the crumbled bacon and tomato.
2. Place all dressing ingredients in a blender
and puree until smooth.
3. Serve dressing drizzled over or on the side.

Makes 1 serving

Egg Salad in Lettuce Wraps

Ingredients
2 large eggs, hard boiled and peeled
Salt and pepper to taste
1 Tablespoon mashed ripe avocado
1 tsp. minced red onion
Dash hot sauce
2 large lettuce leaves such as Boston or leaf
lettuce

Directions
1. In a small bowl combine the eggs, salt,
pepper, avocado, onion and hot sauce and
mash until chunky using the back of a fork.
2. Place the leaves flat on a work surface.
Spoon the egg salad down the middle of each
leaf and carefully fold up the stem end. Roll
to enclose and serve immediately.

Makes 1 serving

Creamed Tuna

Ingredients
1 (5 oz.) can tuna, drained
½ small celery stick, roughly chopped
½ small onion, roughly chopped
¼ medium avocado, diced
Splash almond milk
Salt and pepper to taste
Dash cayenne pepper

Directions
1. Place all ingredients in a food processor and pulse until smooth.
2. Transfer to a bowl and use as a spread or dip.

Makes 1 serving

Seared Jalapeno Tuna Bites

Ingredients
4 oz. ahi tuna fillet cut into 1-inch cubes
Blackened seasoning or Cajun spice mix
2 tsp. olive oil
¼ cup pickled jalapeno slices, drained

Directions
1. Generously sprinkle the seasoning mix over the tuna cubes and set aside.
2. Heat a medium nonstick skillet over high heat and add the oil. Quickly sear the tuna cubes in the hot pan, just until the outsides are browned but the insides are still raw. Remove from the pan and set aside on a serving plate.
3. Add the jalapeno slices to the hot pan and swirl to warm. Pour over the tuna bites and serve.

Makes 1 serving

Steak, Onion, and Carrot Wrap

Ingredients
1 tsp. olive oil
1 (4 oz.) sirloin or beef tenderloin steak
Salt and pepper to taste
1 medium onion, thinly sliced
1 tsp. chopped fresh thyme leaves
1 Tablespoon balsamic vinegar
½ cup grated carrot
3 large lettuce leaves, such as Boston or leaf
lettuce

Directions
1. Heat the oil in a nonstick skillet over high.
Season the beef with salt and pepper and
sear both sides until nicely browned. Cover,
reduce the heat to low, and continue to cook
to desired doneness, about 5 minutes for
medium rare. Transfer steak to a cutting
board and allow to rest.
2. Return the skillet to the heat and add the
onion slices. Season with salt and pepper and
cook, stirring, until softened, about 4
minutes. Add the thyme and cook a further
minute. Remove from the heat and stir in the
vinegar.

(continued on next page)

3. Place the lettuce leaves on a work surface. Slice the steak thinly and place down the middle of the leaves. Top with the onion mixture and a sprinkle of the carrot. Fold up the stem end and roll the leaf to enclose. Serve immediately.

Makes 1 serving

Berry Chicken Salad

Ingredients
2 to 3 cups mixed salad greens
1 cup berries, such as raspberries,
blackberries, or blueberries
1 (4 oz) boneless chicken breast, grilled and
sliced
2 Tablespoons raspberry vinegar
1 Tablespoon olive oil
1 tsp. mustard
1 tsp. agave nectar or honey
Salt and pepper to taste
2 Tablespoons toasted walnuts

Directions
1. In a salad bowl combine the greens, 2/3
cup of the berries, and the chicken slices.
2. In a mini food processor combine the
remaining berries, vinegar, oil, mustard,
agave, salt, and pepper. Pulse until well
combined and pour over the salad. Toss
gently to coat and top with the walnuts
before serving.

Makes 1 serving

Lemon Pepper Tuna Avocado Cups

Ingredients
1 large avocado halved and seeded
½ lemon
1 large egg, hard boiled and peeled
1 (5 oz.) can tuna, drained
1 Tablespoon minced onion
1 Tablespoon minced celery
Salt to taste
Freshly ground black pepper (at least ¼ tsp.)
1 tsp. chopped fresh parsley

Directions
1. Carefully scoop out a small amount of flesh from each avocado half, keeping about ¼-inch still in the peel and transfer to a bowl. Drizzle a little lemon juice over the cut halves and set aside in 2 individual serving bowls.
2. Add the remaining ingredients to the bowl with the avocado, except for the parsley and using the back of a fork or masher, combine until smooth but slightly chunky. Stir in the remaining lemon juice.

(continued on next page)

3. Scoop the mixture into the avocado halves and neatly form a mound. Sprinkle with the parsley and serve immediately.

Makes 2 servings

Steak and Egg Salad

Ingredients
2 to 3 cups baby arugula or spinach
4 oz. steamed asparagus spears
Salt and pepper to taste
Olive oil and lemon juice to taste
2 to 3 oz. grilled beef steak, sliced thin
1 poached egg
1 tsp. chopped fresh basil

Directions
1. Distribute the arugula on a large serving dish. Place the asparagus spears in the middle, season with salt and pepper and drizzle the olive oil and lemon juice over all.
2. Place the sliced beef around the edges of the platter and position the poached egg in the center. Sprinkle the basil over and more pepper if desired.

Makes 1 serving

Steak Apple Kale Salad

Ingredients
2 to 3 cups baby kale
Drizzle of olive oil
Splash apple cider vinegar
Salt and pepper to taste
1 small apple, cored and sliced
1 Tablespoon raisins or currants
1 (4 oz.) beef steak, grilled or broiled, and
sliced

Directions
1. Place kale on a large serving dish, add oil,
vinegar, salt, and pepper, and toss to
combine.
2. Place the apple slices decoratively around
the edges and sprinkle the raisins over.
3. Mound the sliced steak in the middle,
season with ground pepper and serve.

Makes 1 serving

Sweet & Salty Honey Macadamia Nut Salad

Ingredients

For the Nuts:
1 cup roughly chopped salted macadamia
nuts
1 egg white, slightly beaten
¼ cup honey
Dash cinnamon

For the Salad:
2 cups shredded cabbage
1 cup grated carrot
1 Tablespoon olive oil
¼ cup white balsamic vinegar
2 Tablespoons honey
Salt and pepper to taste

Directions
1. Preheat the oven to 300 degrees F. Line a
rimmed baking sheet with parchment paper.
2. In a medium bowl combine the nut
ingredients and stir well. Spread out onto
the parchment and bake for 20 to 25
minutes, stirring occasionally, until nut
coating is crisp and golden.

(continued on next page)

Remove from oven and set aside to cool.
3. In a large bowl toss together the cabbage and carrot. In a small bowl whisk together the oil, vinegar, honey, salt and pepper. Pour over the cabbage mixture and toss well to coat. Stir in the cooled nuts and serve.

Makes 4 to 8 servings

Acorn Squash Soup

Ingredients
2 medium acorn squash
Olive oil for brushing
Salt and pepper to taste
Drizzle honey or maple syrup
1 cup almond milk, warmed
Dash ground nutmeg

Directions
1. Preheat the oven to 375 degrees F. Line a rimmed baking sheet with foil.
2. Cut the squash into halves and scoop out the seeds. Brush the cut flesh lightly with oil and season with salt and pepper. Place cut side down on the pan and bake until squash is slightly tender, about 30 minutes.
3. Flip halves over and drizzle honey on top. Return to oven and continue to bake until very soft and lightly browned. Remove from oven and allow to cool somewhat.
4. Scoop flesh into a food processor or blender and add the almond milk. Puree until smooth and serve warm with a dash of nutmeg on top.

Makes 2 to 4 servings

Roasted Peppers and Veggies in a Meat Wrap

Ingredients
8 oz. sliced roast beef or turkey breast
(medium thick)
Salt and pepper to taste
1 cup roasted red pepper strips or pimentos
2 cups assorted grilled vegetables such as
zucchini or asparagus

Directions
1. Lay meat slices flat on a work surface,
short end facing you, and season with salt
and pepper.
2. Place pepper strips and veggies on end
closest to you (okay if vegetables overhang)
and roll securely to form a "wrap." Warm or
serve chilled.

Makes 2 servings

SNACKS AND SIDE DISHES

Itty Bitty Cucumber Sliders

Ingredients
1 seedless cucumber, unpeeled and sliced
into ¼-inch rounds
Salt to taste
4 oz. ground lamb or beef
Dash curry powder
Fresh ground pepper
Fresh mint leaves
Coconut cream, whipped for serving

Directions
1. Place cucumber slices on paper towels and
salt lightly. Set aside.
2. In a small bowl combine lamb, curry
powder, salt and pepper to taste, and form
into 1-inch wide balls.
3. Heat a nonstick skillet over high heat and
place the lamb balls in a single layer. As they
cook, flatten them with a spatula and
continue browning on both sides until no
longer pink, about 6 minutes. Remove from
pan and set aside to drain.

(continued on next page)

4. Pat dry the cucumber slices and place several on a plate. Top with the mini burgers, fresh mint, and a small dollop of the cream, and place another cucumber slice on top. Serve immediately.

Makes 1 to 2 servings

Beef Stuffed Avocado Cups

Ingredients
2 avocados
1 pound grass-fed ground beef
1/2 cup diced tomatoes
1 Tablespoon lime juice
1 Tablespoon hamburger seasoning

Directions
1. Place ground beef in a non-stick pan and sprinkle with hamburger seasoning. Cook over medium heat until beef is cooked through and brown.
2. Slice the avocados into halves and remove the pits. Scoop out the avocado meat and mash in a large bowl, making sure not to mash too much, leaving large lumps of avocado. Add the tomatoes and lime juice and stir thoroughly.
3. Pour the cooked ground beef into the bowl with the mashed avocado and mix well.
4. Scoop the beef and avocado mixture into the avocado shells. Serve.

Servings: Makes 4 Beef Stuffed Avocado Cups

Pan Fried Sweet Potato

Ingredients
1 medium sweet potato
Salt and pepper to taste
Dash ground cinnamon
Coconut oil for frying
Drizzle of maple syrup

Directions
1. Peel and cut off ends of sweet potato. Slice into ¼-inch medallions. Season with salt, pepper, and cinnamon and set aside.
2. Melt enough coconut oil in a large nonstick skillet to just cover the bottom. Fry the medallions until they are fork tender and lightly browned, about 3 minutes per side. Transfer to a paper towel lined plate to drain.
3. Just before serving, drizzle with a little maple syrup.

Makes 2 servings

Avocado Bacon Dip

Ingredients
1 medium avocado, peeled, seeded and diced
Juice of ½ lime
1 small tomato, diced
1 Tablespoon minced onion
Dash hot sauce
Salt and pepper to taste
3 bacon strips fried to crisp and crumbled

Directions
1. Combine all ingredients in a medium bowl and mash to desired consistency. Serve with vegetables for dipping or as a topping for grilled meats and poultry.

Makes 2 to 4 servings

Peach Salsa

Ingredients
3 medium-size ripe peaches
½ cup finely chopped sweet onion such as
Vidalia
1 small jalapeno pepper, minced
2 Tablespoons lime juice
Salt and pepper to taste
1 Tablespoon chopped fresh cilantro leaves

Directions
1. Bring a pot of water to a bowl. Submerge
peaches in boiling water for 30 to 45 seconds.
Transfer with a slotted spoon to a bowl of ice
water to cool.
2. Using a sharp paring knife, carefully pull
away the peach skins. Halve, removed pits,
and cut flesh into ½-inch dice. Transfer to a
medium bowl.
3. Add the remaining ingredients and toss
gently. Refrigerate or serve immediately.

Makes about 6 servings

Crab & Shrimp Stuffed Mushrooms

Ingredients
6 large white "stuffing" mushroom caps
1 Tablespoon olive oil
Salt and pepper to taste
½ cup crabmeat, picked over
6 large cooked and peeled shrimp, chopped
1 tsp. lemon juice
Dash hot sauce
2 Tablespoons finely chopped nuts

Directions
1. Remove any stems from the caps and wipe clean. Heat the oil in a large nonstick skillet and add the mushroom caps. Season with salt and pepper and turn to brown evenly. Mushrooms should be crisp tender. Set aside on a foil lined baking sheet.
2. In a small bowl combine the crabmeat, shrimp, lemon juice, and hot sauce. Season to taste with salt and pepper. Spoon the mixture evenly into each mushroom cap and top each with the nuts.

(continued on next page)

3. Place under a broiler and heat until the nuts begin to brown and the filling is just warmed through. Serve immediately.

Makes 1 serving

Deviled Eggs

Ingredients
4 large eggs, hard boiled and peeled
Salt and pepper to taste
2 Tablespoons mashed ripe avocado
½ tsp. mustard
1 tsp. pickle relish
Dash paprika

Directions
1. Halve the eggs and scoop the yolks into a small mixing bowl.
2. Add the salt, pepper, avocado, mustard, and relish to the egg yolks and mash well until combined.
3. Spoon into the cooked whites and sprinkle with paprika before serving.

Makes 2 servings

Roasted Red Pepper Dip

Ingredients
1 large red bell pepper
1 large garlic clove
2 tsp. olive oil
Splash balsamic vinegar
Salt and pepper to taste

Directions
1. Place the pepper over an open flame or on a grill and blacken the skin, turning often. Put in a small brown paper bag and allow to steam and cool for 15 minutes.
2. Remove the charred skin from the pepper with a paper towel. Halve the pepper, stem, core, and remove seeds. Chop roughly and add to a food processor.
3. Add the remaining ingredients to the processor and puree until smooth. Taste for seasoning and transfer to a dipping bowl. Serve with raw vegetables.

Makes 2 servings

Onion Steak Bites

Ingredients
1 (4 oz.) sirloin or beef tenderloin steak
Salt and pepper to taste
1 tsp. olive oil
1 medium sweet onion, such as Vidalia
1 tsp. chopped fresh chives

Directions
1. Heat a medium nonstick skillet over high heat. Season the steak with salt and pepper; add the oil to the pan, and brown beef on both sides.
2. Cover, reduce the heat to low, and continue to cook to desired doneness, about 5 minutes for medium rare, depending on thickness.
3. Meanwhile peel and slice the onion into circles to serve as a "cracker" bed and set aside on a serving plate.
4. When steak is cooked, transfer to a board to rest for at least 5 minutes. Slice thinly into strips and mound on the onion crackers. Sprinkle the chives over and serve.

Makes 1 to 2 servings

Turkey Wrapped Pineapple Bites

Ingredients
1 cup cubed fresh pineapple
4 oz. sliced turkey breast
Dash cayenne pepper
1 Tablespoon prepared mustard
1 tsp. maple syrup
Toothpicks to secure

Directions
1. Preheat the oven to 325 degrees F. Line a baking sheet with foil.
2. Wrap each pineapple cube with a turkey slice into a small enclosed package and secure with a toothpick. Place on the prepared sheet and sprinkle with the cayenne.
3. Bake in the oven just until warmed, about 8 minutes.
4. In a small bowl combine the mustard and maple syrup and serve as a dipping sauce.

Makes 1 to 2 servings

Coconutty Crab Dip

Ingredients
4 oz. crabmeat, picked over
Salt and pepper to taste
Splash coconut milk
Dash paprika
1 Tablespoon shredded coconut

Directions
1. In a small bowl carefully combine the crabmeat, salt, pepper, coconut milk, and paprika. Transfer to a small baking dish or medium ramekin and top with the coconut.
2. Place under a broiler just until coconut begins to toast and crab mixture warms, 3 to 5 minutes. Serve with vegetables for dipping.

Makes 2 servings

Crab Puffs

Ingredients
4 oz. crabmeat, picked over
Dash Old Bay Seasoning
Salt and pepper to taste
4 large eggs
2 Tablespoons water
½ tsp. chopped fresh dill
½ tsp. chopped fresh cilantro

Directions
1. Preheat the oven to 325 degrees F. Lightly oil the middle 4 spaces of a standard 12 cup muffin tin.
2. In a medium bowl carefully toss together the crabmeat, Old Bay, salt, and pepper. In another bowl beat together the eggs, water, and herbs. Add the egg mixture to the crab mixture and gently stir to combine.
3. Spoon the mixture into the prepared muffin cups and bake until a toothpick inserted in the middle comes out clean and the tops are lightly browned, 8 to 12 minutes.

(continued on next page)

4. Remove from oven and allow to cool for 2 minutes before removing and serving.

Makes 2 to 4 servings

Cool Salmon Salad Bites

Ingredients
1 6 oz. can wild salmon
1/2 Tablespoon olive oil
1/4 cup diced tomatoes
1/4 cup diced celery
1/4 cup diced green onion
Lemon pepper seasoning to taste
12 slices of cucumber

Directions
1. Mix all ingredients, except the cucumber
slices, in a bowl.
2. Top cucumber slices with salmon salad.
Serve cold.

Servings: Makes 12 Cool Salmon Salad Bites

Pineapple Salsa

Ingredients
1 cup diced pineapple
1/4 cup chopped cucumber
1 Tablespoon minced shallots
1/4 cup chopped bell pepper
2 Tablespoons chopped cilantro
1 tsp. sea salt
1 tsp. ground black pepper
1 1/2 Tablespoons lime juice
1 Tablespoon lemon juice
1 Tablespoon minced jalapeño

Directions
1. Mix all ingredients in a bowl. Refrigerate for at least 1 hour. Serve.

Servings: 4

Salty Sweet Potato Chips

Ingredients
2 medium sweet potatoes
2 Tablespoons olive oil
Sea salt and pepper to taste

Directions
1. Preheat oven to 200 degrees.
2. Slice the sweet potatoes thinly. Place on baking sheet lined with wax paper and drizzle with olive oil. Make sure none of the sweet potato slices are overlapping. Sprinkle with salt and pepper.
3. Bake for 2 hours or until slightly brown. The sweet potato chips crisp up once cooled.

Servings: 3

Fall Festival Apple Chips

Ingredients
2 medium apples
1 1/2 Tablespoons maple syrup
1/2 Tablespoon water
1 1/2 tsp. cinnamon
1/2 tsp. ground black pepper

Directions
1. Preheat oven to 200 degrees.
2. In a bowl, mix together maple syrup,
water, cinnamon, and ground black pepper.
Core apples and thinly slice them. Set them
on a baking sheet lined with wax paper,
making sure none overlap.
3. Use a pastry brush to brush the syrup
mixture onto the apple slices.
4. Bake for 2 hours or until browned and
allow to cool before serving. The apple chips
crisp up once cooled.

Servings: 3

Spicy Garlic Broccoli

Ingredients
4 cups broccoli florets
1 Tablespoon olive oil
2 Tablespoons minced shallots
1 Tablespoon minced garlic
1 Tablespoon lemon juice
1 tsp. ground black pepper
1 tsp. crushed red pepper

Directions
1. Toss all the ingredients into a large, non-stick pan.
2. Cook over medium heat for 10 minutes, or until broccoli florets are tender.

Servings: 4

Bacon Wrapped Apple Bites

Ingredients
1 apple
4 slices of bacon

Directions
1. Put the bacon in a non-stick pan and set to medium heat. Heat for about 10 minutes or until bacon is a deep brown color.
2. Slice the apple into eight slices.
3. While the bacon is still warm and pliable, tear into eight pieces and wrap each bacon piece around an apple slice. Secure with toothpicks. Serve.

Servings: 4

Bacon Wrapped Avocado Bites

Ingredients:
1 ripe, but firm avocado
4 slices of bacon
Sea salt and pepper to taste

Directions:
1. Put the bacon in a non-stick pan and set to medium heat. Heat for about 10 minutes or until bacon is a deep brown color.
2. Slice the avocado into eight slices. Sprinkle salt and pepper on the avocado slices.
3. While the bacon is still warm and pliable, tear into eight pieces and wrap each bacon piece around an avocado slice. Secure with toothpicks. Serve.

Servings: 4

Beef Stuffed Sweet Potatoes

Ingredients
1 pound grass-fed ground beef
1 Tablespoon hamburger seasoning
4 medium sweet potatoes
2 Tablespoons minced shallots
1 Tablespoon minced garlic
3 Tablespoons olive oil

Directions
1. Preheat oven to 375.
2. Place sweet potatoes on a baking sheet and bake in preheated oven for 1 hour. Remove the sweet potatoes from the oven and allow to cool enough to handle.
3. While the sweet potatoes are cooling, pour olive oil, shallots, and garlic into a pan and heat over medium heat until bubbling.
4. Place ground beef in a non-stick pan and sprinkle with hamburger seasoning. Cook over medium heat until beef is cooked through and brown.
5. Scoop the sweet potato meat from the shells and pour into a large bowl. Mash the sweet potatoes well. Stir in cooked ground beef and the shallot and garlic mixture. Stir.

(continued on next page)

6. Scoop the sweet potato and beef mixture into the sweet potato shells. Serve.

Servings: 4

DINNER

Nutty Blueberry Burgers

Ingredients
1/2 cup finely chopped macadamia nuts
1 pound grass-fed ground beef
1 cup blueberries
1 Tablespoon hamburger seasoning

Directions
1. Mix together ground beef, blueberries, nuts, and hamburger seasoning in a large bowl.
2. Mash the beef mixture into four patties using your hands.
3. Heat on a non-stick pan over medium heat for 5 minutes, then flip the patties and cook for an additional 5 minutes.
4. Optionally, top with blueberries and nuts. Serve.

Servings: 4

Spicy Apple Maple Bacon Burgers

Ingredients
1 cup diced apple
1 pound grass-fed ground beef
1 Tablespoon hamburger seasoning
2 Tablespoons maple syrup
8 slices of cooked bacon
1 sliced and seeded jalapeño

Directions
1. Mix together ground beef, apples, maple syrup, cooked bacon, and hamburger seasoning in a large bowl.
2. Mash the beef mixture into four patties using your hands.
3. Heat on a non-stick pan over medium heat for 5 minutes, then flip the patties and cook for an additional 5 minutes.
4. Top with jalapeño slices. Serve.

Servings: 4

Bacon & Egg Burgers

Ingredients
4 eggs
1 pound grass-fed ground beef
1 Tablespoon hamburger seasoning
8 slices of cooked bacon

Directions
1. Mash beef into four patties using your hands. Place ground beef patties in a non-stick pan and sprinkle with hamburger seasoning. Cook over medium heat until beef is cooked through and brown.
2. While the beef patties are cooking, cook the eggs over medium heat on a non-stick skillet until over-easy.
3. Top burger patties with two slices of bacon each and one egg. Serve.

Servings: 4

Roasted Blueberries Over Salmon

Ingredients
2 medium salmon fillets
1 cup blueberries
1/4 cup chopped walnuts

Directions
1. Preheat oven to 375.
2. Place salmon fillets on a baking sheet. Top with blueberries and walnuts.
3. Bake in oven for 20 minutes. Serve.

Servings: 2

Sizzling Garlic Salmon

Ingredients
2 medium salmon fillets
2 Tablespoons fresh chopped garlic
1/4 cup olive oil
1 Tablespoon crushed red pepper

Directions
1. Preheat oven to 400.
2. Place salmon fillets in an oven-safe bowl.
3. In a small bowl, mix the garlic, olive oil, and crushed red pepper.
4. Pour olive oil mixture over salmon fillets.
5. Bake in oven for 16 minutes, flipping once halfway between cooking. Serve.

Servings: 2

Honey Apple Smoked Salmon

Ingredients
2 medium smoked salmon fillets
1 cup diced apple
1 Tablespoon honey
1/4 tsp. ground black pepper
1/4 tsp. cinnamon

Directions
1. Preheat oven to 375.
2. Place salmon fillets on a baking sheet.
3. Toss apples, honey, pepper, and cinnamon over salmon fillets.
4. Bake in oven for 20 minutes. Serve.

Servings: 2

Fish Nachos with Pineapple Salsa

Ingredients
2 halibut fillets
1 Tablespoon minced garlic
1 Tablespoon minced shallots
1/2 tsp. lemon juice
1 diced avocado
1/2 cup chopped romaine lettuce
1 cup Pineapple Salsa (Recipe included in this book)
1 cup Salty Sweet Potato Chips (Recipe included in this book)

Directions
1. Preheat oven to 350.
2. Chop the halibut fillets into small pieces and toss into a bowl. Add garlic, shallots, and lemon to the bowl and stir thoroughly.
3. Place the halibut fillets on a baking sheet. Bake halibut fillets for 9 minutes.
4. On serving plate, put down a layer of salty sweet potato chips. Place the halibut fillets on top of the chips.
5. Top the fillets with pineapple salsa, romaine lettuce, and avocado. Serve.

Servings: 2

Lemon Mousse Over Fish

Ingredients
8 oz. firm fleshed fish, grilled, baked or broiled

For Mousse:
½ cup chicken or vegetable broth
1 large egg
2 Tablespoons lemon juice
Salt and pepper to taste
2 Tablespoons coconut cream

Directions
1. While fish is cooking, prepare mousse. Heat broth in a small saucepan just to boiling then set aside.
2. In a medium bowl whisk the egg until frothy. Add lemon juice, salt and pepper, and whisk until well combined. Slowly pour in broth while continuing to whisk, then pour back into saucepan.
3. Cook mixture over low heat, whisking gently, until thickened, 8 to 10 minutes.

(continued on next page)

4. In a small bowl whisk coconut cream until just thickened, then fold into egg mixture. Immediately serve over fish.

Makes 2 servings

Turkey Spinach Meatballs

Ingredients
1 (10 oz.) pkg frozen chopped spinach
1 lb. ground turkey
1 large egg white
Pinch dried herbs
Salt and pepper to taste
2 Tablespoons olive oil
Juice ½ lemon

Directions
1. Cook spinach according to package directions. Cool slightly then squeeze out all excess liquid. Set spinach aside to cool completely.
2. In a large bowl combine spinach, turkey, egg white, herbs, salt and pepper.
3. Heat oil in a large nonstick skillet over medium high heat. Form turkey mixture into 16 meatballs and sauté in the oil, turning occasionally to brown completely. Add lemon juice, reduce heat to low, and cover.
4. Cook until meatballs are no longer pink inside, about 8 minutes. Serve immediately with more lemon if desired.

Makes 4 servings

Margarita Fish Enchiladas

Ingredients
2 (4 oz) fillets flounder or sole
Salt and pepper to taste
Dash chili powder
Dash ground cumin
Juice 1 lime
2 Tablespoons fresh tomato salsa

Directions
1. Season both sides of the fillets with salt, pepper, chili powder, and cumin. Squeeze a little lime juice over the "skin" side.
2. Divide salsa and place down middle of "skin" side of each fillet. Carefully fold over each end to enclose. Squeeze more lime juice over top.
3. Place enchiladas on a flame-proof pan and broil until flesh begins to flake, about 5 minutes. Transfer to a serving plate and drizzle remaining lime juice over.

Makes 1 or 2 servings

Coconut Fried Scallops

Ingredients
½ cup shredded coconut
½ tsp. grated orange zest
2 Tablespoons coconut flour
Salt and pepper to taste
8 oz. sea scallops
Coconut oil for frying

Directions
1. In a shallow dish combine the coconut, orange zest, coconut flour, salt, and pepper.
2. Pat dry the scallops and dredge in the coconut mixture. Set aside on a wire rack.
3. Heat enough oil in a heavy skillet to come ¼ inch up the sides. Heat to 365 degrees or until a pinch of coconut sizzles when added.
4. Carefully place the coated scallops in the hot oil and fry until golden, about 1 minute per side. Drain on paper towels and serve immediately.

Makes 2 servings

Nut Crusted Tilapia

Ingredients
4 oz. tilapia fillets
Salt and pepper to taste
1 Tablespoon chopped almonds or pecans
Drizzle coconut oil
1 tsp. maple syrup

Directions
1. Preheat the oven to 350 degrees F.
2. Place fillets on a foil lined baking sheet and sprinkle with salt and pepper.
3. In a small bowl combine chopped nuts, oil, and maple syrup. Press onto top of tilapia and bake until fish begins to flake and crust is lightly browned, about 12 minutes.

Makes 1 serving

Pepper Stuffed Burgers

Ingredients
1 lb. ground beef or turkey
Salt and pepper to taste
1 Tablespoon chopped fresh basil
1 cup roasted pepper strips or pimentos
Splash balsamic vinegar or red wine

Directions
1. Divide the ground meat into 8 equal
mounds and shape into thin patties.
2. In a small bowl stir together roasted
peppers, basil, salt, and pepper. Divide the
pepper mixture into 4 and mound each
portion onto one burger patty, pressing down
gently. Top each mounded patty with a plain
patty and carefully seal the edges together
by pressing without changing the shape.
2. Heat a large nonstick skillet and season
the burgers with additional salt and pepper.
Fry until nicely browned to desired doneness,
about 4 minutes per side for medium.
Remove burgers and add vinegar to hot
skillet. Swirl and pour over each cooked
burger before serving.

Makes 4 servings

Stuffed Green Peppers

Ingredients
2 medium green bell peppers
1 Tablespoon olive oil
1 small onion, minced
1 garlic clove, minced
Salt and pepper to taste
½ lb. lean ground beef
1 (8 oz.) can tomato sauce
¼ cup water
Dash ground allspice

Directions
1. Bring a pot of salted water large enough to hold the peppers to a boil.
2. Meanwhile, in a nonstick skillet heat the oil over high heat and add the onion and garlic. Sprinkle with salt and pepper and cook, stirring often, until lightly browned, about 2 minutes. Add the beef and break apart with a fork. Cook, stirring occasionally, until meat is no longer pink, about 4 minutes.

(continued on next page)

3. Stir in the tomato sauce, water, and allspice, bring to a simmer, and continue to cook for 5 minutes. Set aside. Preheat the oven to 350 degrees F.

4. Submerge the peppers in the boiling water and blanch until crisp tender, about 5 minutes. Drain and cool slightly. Cut off the tops of the peppers and scoop out the seeds and membrane. Stuff each pepper with the beef filling and place the caps on top. Snuggle into a baking dish and bake until the peppers are fork tender and the filling is bubbly, about 25 minutes.

Makes 2 servings

Bacon Wrapped Garlic Scallops

Ingredients
6 large sea scallops
Salt and pepper to taste
3 strips of bacon, halved
2 tsp. olive oil
2 garlic cloves sliced
1 Tablespoon maple syrup or agave nectar
Toothpicks to secure

Directions
1. Preheat the oven to 400 degrees F. Line a rimmed baking pan with foil.
2. Pat dry the scallops and season with salt and pepper. Wrap each scallop around its edge with a bacon strip half and secure with a toothpick. Bake in the oven until the scallops are no longer opaque and the bacon has begun to crisp, about 8 minutes. Remove from the pan and drain on paper towels. Keep warm.
3. In a small nonstick skillet heat the olive oil over medium heat. Add the garlic slices, season with salt and lightly brown, about 1 minute. Remove from the heat, stir in the maple syrup and spoon over the scallops before serving.

Makes 1 serving

Jalapeno Mango Chicken

Ingredients
1/2 mango, peeled, seeded and diced
1 small jalapeno pepper, minced
1 Tablespoon olive oil
Juice of 1 lime
¼ tsp. ground cumin
8 oz. boneless, skinless chicken breasts
Salt and pepper to taste
1 Tablespoon chopped cilantro

Directions
1. In a blender combine the mango, jalapeno, olive oil, lime, and cumin and puree until smooth. Place the chicken in a shallow bowl and pour the mixture over. Turn to coat, cover, and marinate in the refrigerator for 1 hour or more.
2. Heat an indoor or outdoor grill. Season the chicken with salt and pepper and grill over medium-high heat until no longer pink inside and an internal read thermometer registers 165 degrees.
3. Place chicken on serving plates and sprinkle with the cilantro.

Makes 2 servings

Halibut Under Mango Salsa

Ingredients
2 halibut fillets or steaks
Salt and pepper to taste
Dash paprika
1 mango, peeled, seeded, and diced small
½ medium red onion, diced
1 medium tomato, seeded and diced
1 small jalapeno, minced
Juice of ½ lime
Drizzle of olive oil
2 tsp. chopped cilantro

Directions
1. Season the fillets with salt, pepper, and paprika and set aside. Heat an indoor or outdoor grill to medium-high.
2. Combine the remaining ingredients in a bowl and gently toss to combine. Taste for the addition of salt and pepper and set aside.
3. Grill the halibut until no longer opaque and the flesh begins to flake, 3 to 4 minutes per side, depending on thickness.
4. Transfer each fillet to a serving plate and mound half the mango salsa onto each one.

Makes 2 servings

Jalapeno Mushroom "Burger"

Ingredients
2 Portobello mushroom caps
Salt and pepper to taste
Oil for drizzling
4 oz. ground beef or turkey
1 Tablespoon pickled jalapeno, chopped
2 sundried tomatoes, chopped
Pinch dried herbs
Mustard, shaved onion, sliced tomato, and
lettuce for serving

Directions
1. Using a tsp., scrape out the black gills of
the mushroom cap and wipe clean with a
damp cloth. Season with salt and pepper and
drizzle with olive oil. Set aside.
2. In a small bowl mix together the beef,
jalapeno, sundried tomatoes, herbs, and salt
and pepper to taste. Form into a burger and
set aside.
3. Heat an indoor or outdoor grill to medium
high and grill the mushroom caps just until
slightly fork tender. Grill the burger to
desired doneness, about 5 minutes per side
for medium.

(continued on next page)

4. Place the cooked burger on top of one of the caps, add the mustard, onion, tomato, and lettuce and finish with the remaining mushroom cap. Serve as a "burger" with plenty of napkins!

Makes 1 serving

Coconut Lime Margarita Chicken

Ingredients
2 tsp. coconut oil
2 boneless, skinless chicken breasts, diced
Salt and pepper to taste
1 shallot, minced
Juice of 1 lime
½ cup chicken broth
¼ cup coconut cream

Directions
1. Melt coconut oil in a large nonstick pan.
Season diced chicken with salt and pepper
and brown in oil without cooking through.
Transfer with a slotted spoon to a clean bowl.
2. Add shallot to pan and cook until softened,
about 2 minutes. Add lime juice and broth
and bring to a simmer. Put chicken with
juices back into pan and simmer until cooked
through, about 3 minutes.
3. Whisk in coconut cream off of heat, taste
for additional seasoning, and serve.

Makes 2 servings

Tuna with Coconut Mousse

Ingredients
1 (4 oz) ahi tuna steak
Salt and pepper to taste
Juice of 1/2 lime
¼ cup coconut cream
1 Tablespoon toasted flaked coconut

Directions
1. Season the tuna with salt and pepper and grill on an indoor or outdoor barbecue to desired doneness, about 3 minutes per side for medium. Transfer to a plate and drizzle with the lime juice.
2. In a small bowl whisk the coconut cream until it thickens. Dollop on the tuna steak and sprinkle the toasted coconut over.

Makes 1 serving

Tuna with Avocado Mousse

1 (4 oz) ahi tuna steak
Salt and pepper to taste
Juice of 1/2 lime
2 Tablespoons coconut cream
¼ cup mashed avocado

1. Season the tuna with salt and pepper and grill on an indoor or outdoor barbecue to desired doneness, about 3 minutes per side for medium. Transfer to a plate and drizzle with the lime juice.
2. In a small bowl whisk the coconut cream until it thickens. Fold in the mashed avocado and season with salt and pepper. Dollop on the tuna steak and serve.

Makes 1 serving

Paleo Fiesta Nachos

Ingredients
1 recipe for "Sweet Potato Chips"
1 boneless, skinless chicken breast, grilled
and diced
1 small onion, diced
1 small tomato, seeded and diced
2 Tablespoons pickled jalapeno slices
2 Tablespoons sliced olives
1 cup finely shredded lettuce

Directions
1. Preheat the oven to 375 degrees F. Line a
rimmed baking sheet with foil.
2. Spread out the sweet potato chips, slightly
layering to create a bed. Top with the diced
chicken, onion, tomato, and jalapeno. Bake
until just warmed through, about 8 minutes.
3. Transfer carefully to a serving platter and
sprinkle the olives over. Mound the lettuce in
the middle and serve.

Makes 1 to 2 servings

Sizzling Shrimp in Chili Oil

Ingredients
8 oz raw jumbo shrimp, shelled and deveined
¼ cup chili-infused oil
½ tsp. Cajun or Creole seasoning
1 Tablespoon chopped fresh parsley leaves

Directions
1. Preheat the oven to 400 degrees F.
2. Place the shrimp in a single layer in a shallow gratin dish. Evenly pour the oil over and sprinkle with the seasoning.
3. Roast in the oven until the shrimp is pink and the oil is sizzling, 15 to 20 minutes. Stir occasionally to cook evenly. Just before serving sprinkle with the chopped parsley.

Makes 2 servings

Chicken Fajita Kebabs

Ingredients
8 oz. boneless, skinless chicken breast, cubed
Salt and pepper to taste
1 tsp. chili powder
½ tsp. ground cumin
1 large green pepper, cored, seeded and cut
into squares
1 medium sweet onion, peeled and cut into
wedges
Oil for grilling

Directions
1. Season the cubed chicken with salt,
pepper, chili powder and cumin. Thread,
alternating with the green pepper and onion,
onto skewers and set aside.
2. Heat an indoor or outdoor grill to medium
high and cook the kebabs, turning
frequently, until the chicken is no longer
pink and the vegetables are crisp tender,
about 8 minutes. Serve immediately.

Makes 2 servings

DESSERTS

Syrupy Strawberry Banana Delight

Ingredients
1 banana
1/2 cup sliced strawberries
1/2 tsp. cinnamon
1/2 tsp. pumpkin pie spice
1/2 Tablespoon maple syrup
1 Tablespoon crushed pecans

Directions
1. Make a long slit across the top of the
banana. Fill with strawberries.
2. Top with cinnamon, pumpkin pie spice,
maple syrup, and crushed pecans. Serve.

Servings: 1

Maple Roasted Peaches

Ingredients
1 peach
1 Tablespoon maple syrup
2 Tablespoons chopped walnuts
1 tsp. cinnamon

Directions
1. Preheat oven to 375.
2. Slice peach in half and remove pit. Set peaches, cut side up, on a baking sheet. Drizzle syrup, walnuts, and cinnamon over peaches. Bake for 15 minutes. Serve.

Servings: 2

Orange Bomb

Ingredients
1 large navel orange
2 ice cubes
2 tsp. fresh mint leaves
1 tsp. agave nectar or honey

Directions
1. Halve the orange and scoop out all flesh into a food processor or blender, discarding any seeds. Place empty halves in freezer.
2. Add remaining ingredients to orange pieces and process until frosty and snow-like. Transfer mixture into frozen empty halves and serve or keep frozen.

Makes 1 or 2 servings

Mint Watermelon Ice

Ingredients
2 cups cubed watermelon, seeds discarded
4 ice cubes
1 tsp. lemon juice
1 Tablespoon agave nectar
Coarse sea salt

Directions
1. Combine all ingredients except the salt in a food processor or blender. Pulse or grate until frosty and snow-like.
2. Transfer to 2 serving dishes and sprinkle with a little sea salt before serving.

Makes 2 servings

Banana Ice Cream with Syrup and Pecans

Ingredients
1 medium banana, peeled, sliced, and frozen
1/2 cup almond or coconut milk
4 tsp. maple syrup
2 Tablespoons chopped toasted pecans.

Directions
1. Place the frozen banana, almond milk, and 1 tsp. of the syrup in a blender and puree until smooth. Transfer to a serving dish.
2. Pour the remaining syrup over and sprinkle with the pecans.

Makes 1 serving

Coconut Mousse Topped with Berries and Nuts

Ingredients
1 cup coconut cream
2 Tablespoons agave nectar or maple syrup
1 cup diced fresh berries (any type)
¼ cup toasted nuts

Directions
1. Whisk together coconut cream and agave until thickened. Spoon into 2 parfait cups.
2. Top with the berries and nuts, and serve.

Makes 2 servings

Paleo Chocolate Mousse

Ingredients
1 cup thick coconut milk
2 Tablespoons agave nectar or maple syrup
1 Tablespoon cocoa powder
½ tsp. vanilla
½ medium avocado, diced

Directions
1. In a blender or food processor combine all the ingredients except the avocado and process until smooth.
2. Add the avocado and continue processing until thick and creamy. Transfer to a serving dish and chill before serving.

Makes 1 to 2 servings

Peppermint Peach Mousse-Cream

Ingredients
2 medium-size ripe peaches
2 to 3 drops peppermint oil
1 Tablespoon agave nectar or maple syrup
2/3 cup coconut cream

Directions
1. Prepare peaches as instructed in "Peach Salsa" recipe up through #2 directions.
2. Stir in peppermint oil and agave and taste for sweetness. Add more if desired.
3. Transfer mixture to a blender or food processor and puree. Meanwhile, in a medium bowl whisk the coconut cream until thickened.
4. Pour the peach mixture into the cream and gently fold in, not to lose volume. Spoon into servings dishes and chill until ready to serve.

Makes 2 to 4 servings

Strawberries in Chocolate Peppermint Mousse

Ingredients
1 recipe for "Paleo Chocolate Mousse"
1 to 2 drops peppermint oil
1 cup strawberries, whole or diced

Directions
1. Prepare chocolate mousse as directed adding peppermint oil to blender. Transfer to a serving dish and allow to chill.
2. Serve either as a dip for whole strawberries or as a base for diced berries.

Makes 1 to 2 servings

3764539R00067

Printed in Great Britain
by Amazon.co.uk, Ltd.,
Marston Gate.